BUSINESS GUIDE for HE
and PRACTITIONERS of C
ALTERNATIVE MEDICINE

HOW TO FIND WHAT YOU NEED TO KNOW
Second Edition

Manage your practice as a business
Promote the sale of your CAM or therapy products and services
More than 150 links to useful websites

RICHARD EATON LLB
Mentor for new businesses

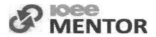

Touchworks Ltd

LinkedIn: uk.linkedin.com/in/richardmceaton
'Owning a Business' website: bit.ly/1REoab
Personal website: www.richardeaton.co.uk

Available online as an ebook from digital stores at:
www.books2read.com/BG4HT

Coil-bound paperback book available from www.lulu.com

DEDICATION

I dedicate this book to my wife, Marion Eaton — a talented lawyer (now retired), a Reiki Master Teacher, marioneaton.co.uk, an author, marioneaton.com, and so many other things that are too numerous to mention here — with my love and thanks for the love, devotion and inspiration that she has given to me and to our daughters for so many years.

ABOUT THE AUTHOR

Richard Eaton has a professional background as a barrister of Lincoln's Inn, now retired, as a lecturer in law and as a business mentor.

He is a director of his own company, Touchworks Ltd, which is engaged in publishing, consultancy, business mentoring and the promotion and supply of complementary medicine training and services. He has acted as a Health & Social Care sector mediator, a lecturer in law delivering law courses at professional, higher and further education levels and as a New Enterprise Network and Start-up Loans Business Mentor. He is a member of the *Institute of Enterprise and Entrepreneurs (MIoEE)*.

For many years, Richard has supported and campaigned for the freedom of practitioners to practise and for their patients to receive Health Therapy and Complementary & Alternative Medicine (CAM) services and products. He formerly owned and practice-managed, jointly with his wife Marion Eaton (a professional aromatherapist and Reiki Master Teacher) *The Professional Centre for Holistic Health*, Old Town, Hastings, East Sussex in South East England. The Centre provided full practising facilities for 16 therapists and CAM Practitioners.

Richard takes a keen interest in the provision and development of CAM and Integrated Healthcare within both the public and the private health sectors.

He is a mentor with the *Passport to Success* scheme

managed by the *University of Brighton* and also a mentor to students of the *Chartered Institute of Legal Executives (CILEX)*. Richard is a participant in the government funded *Get Mentoring* initiative that delivers mentoring to any type of micro, small and medium sized business. He is profiled in the public directory of the online *Get Mentoring NEN Portal*.

In addition to writing this book, Richard has had published articles, discussion documents & research proposals relating to alternative dispute resolution, clinical practice management (complementary medicine), Human Rights and the professional training of legal practitioners. He was a participant in *The Legal Education & Training Report 2013*.

Links to articles written by Richard and published on Positive Health Online, together with links to CAM websites, can be found in the Appendix to this book. Richard writes a quarterly Blog about CAM for the College of Medicine

For more information, see: richardeaton.co.uk

CONTENTS

ABOUT THIS BOOK

This book is about the business aspects of starting and managing a complementary and alternative medicine (CAM) or health therapy practice. It is based on the second edition of the first book in this series titled *Owning a Business: Things you need to Know* (bit.ly/1REoab).

As business owners, Practitioners need to know about the business processes that will define and sustain the success of their practice. So the aim of this book is not to focus on the delivery of treatments and therapies but rather to introduce the Practitioner to the business and management facilities, opportunities and support which can assist them to start, develop and expand their practice.

In addition to treating their clients, many Practitioners engage in the manufacture and retail sale of CAM and therapy products. Accordingly, the scope of this book also includes business suggestions for the promotion and sale of these products.

Although it is primarily aimed at Practitioners practising within the United Kingdom and using UK institutions and websites, many sections of this book should also be relevant to any CAM or therapy practice where ever it is based.

My aim is to present you with a general, brief, simple, easily accessible and straightforward overview of the business processes that could benefit your practice and, should you desire, to enable you to access more detailed information by linking to selected websites.

Throughout, I have, for ease of reference, referred to 'clients' rather than 'patients'. Where you are selling products, you should assume that this also means 'customers'. Where I refer to 'Practitioners' this means Practitioners of a CAM or of a health therapy business, although I appreciate that many Practitioners will consider themselves to be practising within both of these sectors. In the event that any information contained or referred to in this book conflicts with the guidance you receive from your membership organisation or regulator, then such guidance should take precedence and be a matter for your professional judgement

This book does not provide information about the management of finance or the preparation of business accounts but it does contain a section exploring *Sources of Finance* together with web links that will help you to find professional help, including in relation to legal matters, and to access guidance issued by H M Revenue & Customs.

The Appendix to this book contains many links to websites operating from the UK, the United States of America and Europe. By way of example, I have included some website links relating to a selected treatment (homeopathy) and a health condition (cancer). Searching this online information will assist you to research and to compare membership organisations, marketing and pricing strategies, the design of advertising and promotional material and the evidence-base for your practice specialisms.

It is important to adopt the right approach to reading this book. Start by reading it without linking to the websites. Then return to the beginning and read it again, this time linking to the detailed (website) business information that is relevant to your practice. Read it on a 'step by step' basis, reviewing each section in turn. You do not have to remember it all.

If you are proposing to start a practice, it is likely that once you have become self-employed you will never want to be an employee again. Instead, you will appreciate the independence, freedom and flexibility that enables you to control your own business and to avoid the internal politics and rigid bureaucracy that can exist in some employer organisations. The availability of affordable, innovative technology means that it is now easier and cheaper than ever to start and to manage a practice. Owning a business is a challenge that more and more people aspire to. For instance, according to surveys by Enterprise Nation (https://www.enterprisenation.com/), 65% of young people would like to have their own business at some time during their careers.

Purely from a business perspective, your practice is about finding clients and selling your professional services and products to them. I hope that by reading this book you will find this easier to achieve. Even as the owner of an established practice, you may well find yourself returning to it again and again.

Note: While the website links are regularly updated, if a link should fail please google the appropriate keywords.

ACHIEVING SUCCESS

A great deal of useful information is available online. It is just a case of knowing where to find it. Your first task is to establish what information is relevant to your practice. As you read, anticipate how the information that you review will become even more relevant as your business develops. Even at the start of your business, you should be planning for its future over at least the next 2 to 3 years.

Remember, the exciting news is that this is, or will be, your practice. You control and are responsible for meeting the medical, therapy and healthcare expectations of your clients. All of the duties and responsibilities relating to your business will be yours although, as this book indicates, there is help and support available should you wish to use it. Planning your practice properly from the outset will be fundamental to its success.

As a business owner, what qualities do you need to be successful? You need to have an in depth knowledge of the products and services that you supply to your clients. You need to be more than just ambitious. To expand your practice, you must have the vision to see the 'bigger picture' to identify new opportunities, be resilient and able to cope with failure and be proactive, assertive, innovative, creative and prepared to take the initiative. It is important that you constantly monitor the quality and effectiveness of your products or services and show real commitment to your clients, professional colleagues and business contacts. In business, you have to take risks and have the conviction that you are right while being realistic, particularly with regard to the time it will take for your new practice to become financially viable. You will have to work hard and be focused on achieving success but at the same time be willing and able to 'see' your practice through the 'eyes' of your clients. Be prepared to adjust your management style, services and products to meet your clients' needs.

The degree of your success will not only depend on how good you are at working IN your practice but also on how effectively you work ON your business.

There are three basic but essential requirements for achieving success in any business, including in your practice:

1. Undertake a practising specialism that will continue to interest you;

2. Provide services and products which your clients want and which, preferably, are not provided by other Practitioners in your market area (your competitors);

3. Follow a healthy and sustainable work-life balance. Even health Practitioners forget to do this.

It may be sensible, at least initially, to focus your practice activity and its funding and other resources on a 'niche' market for a particular product or service. You can extend the range of these as your practice develops and to reflect changes in your clients' needs.

In business, as with anything, avoid trying to do too much too soon, for instance by launching too many products or services at the same time. This could result in your marketing initiatives and resources being utilised ineffectively, with the result that your clients may become confused and dissatisfied. They need to understand precisely and simply what your practice has to offer and how much it will cost them. Carefully research the requirements of your prospective clients before you invest money in, or take any decisions about, the formation and structure of your practice. Discover what your clients want and the extent to which (if at all) they will be prepared to attend your practice and pay your professional fees. Make sure that they understand the value of what they are buying from you and how you justify the price that you charge for your products and services.

As a smaller business, you have the opportunity to exploit the trading deficiencies of your larger competitors, for example by providing a more personal, flexible and versatile client-focused service than other, larger, health sector providers. Think strategically and assess how you can exploit the strengths and weaknesses of your competitors and how you may make best use your professional skills and business assets.

Aim to achieve a sustainable work-life balance. According to research by the *Federation of Small Businesses*, 69.4% of small business owners set up their business in order to achieve greater freedom and independence in their working life and yet almost 66% of respondents worked more than 46 hours a week, with 44% working between 49 and 60 hours and 22% reporting an average working week of over 60 hours.

The freedom and rewards of running your own practice will be yours to enjoy but you will also need to bear the burden of the restrictions, regulations, losses and failures which most businesses from time to time experience. You need to prepare yourself for all eventualities. Effective business planning and practice management will help you to do this. Be prepared to seek and take good professional advice and realise that it is what you don't want to hear that can sometimes prove to be the most valuable information for your business.

CHOOSING A BUSINESS NAME FOR YOUR PRACTICE

Think carefully about choosing a Business Name which has been defined as: *a name used by any person, partnership or company for carrying on a business, unless it is the same as their own name.*

With regard to your Business Name, ask yourself:

✓ Is it sufficiently memorable? Will my clients easily remember it and is it relevant to what my practice provides?

✓ Is it accessible online and offline, through social media, LinkedIn, my website's domain name and in business and professional directories?

✓ Is it included in my digital marketing?

✓ Does it need legal protection by the registration of words or a logo as a trade mark?

Take legal advice if your practice's name is similar to that of another business and discover whether it requires approval or disclosure further to business names legislation. Check, too, that it does not conflict with a registered Trade Mark. For information about choosing a business name, research: www.gov.uk/choose-company-name.

Remember the importance of your own name. Following a recommendation or referral to you, this may be what a prospective client looks and searches for first. So make sure that it is easily accessible, both online and offline, along with any practice name you adopt

YOUR PRACTISING ADDRESS

For administrative, legal and logistical reasons your practice will need to have a trading ('practising') address. Where this is located will depend on what type of practice you have and where your target market (prospective clients) is located. Much may depend on what private and public transport facilities are available to you and to your clients.

Generally, to practice-manage your business efficiently, you will need to have access to a consistently well lighted, heated, quiet, clean, comfortable and organised work space which is adequate in size and properly served by appropriate technology, business and personal facilities.

If your practice requires you meet with your clients or contacts (other than, for instance, by Skype) or to make presentations to or hold meetings with them (whether as individuals or in a group) then you will need to make arrangements for adequate facilities to be available either at your practising address or at another reputable business venue.

Facilities should also be secure and sufficiently private to enable discussions with and treatment of your clients to be confidential.

You need to be aware of legislation and regulations that apply to your workplace, particularly if you propose to provide workspace for staff, students or an apprentice.

Many practices, like other small businesses, are based at the Practitioner's home. This has obvious implications, including in relation to insurance cover and tax liability, which you should discuss with your Insurance Company and a Chartered Accountant. Research undertaken by the Federation of Small

Businesses (see: http://tinyurl.com/l24rcqc) states as follows:

'The three main reasons why people choose to run a business from home are to contain costs, because it is more convenient and because there is no need for commercial premises. In addition to these factors, the work–life balance that people can achieve by working from home allows them to be close to family and friends. The flipside of the positive experiences that running a home-based business can bring is that difficulties can often arise with things such as space, parking, IT and, of special relevance for work–life balance, the lack of any real boundaries between work and leisure and the encroachment of work onto 'family time.' For women, having no boundaries between work and leisure and work invading family time were also important. As level of turnover and number of employees in the home-based business grow, these issues become steadily more significant.'

According to figures published by the Office for National Statistics, one in ten people work from home. *Home-working* or *Remote-working* can be cheaper and more productive than working in a traditional centralised workplace as it avoids distractions, overheads and time wasted while commuting. It also enables the Practitioner to pace their work thereby reducing work-pressure. Technology facilitates working from home with the use instantaneous communications tools like GoToMeeting, Skype, Citrix, and Google Chat. These could be especially useful for talking-therapies, where a face-to-face consultation is not possible, or when online meetings need to take place, for instance to facilitate training programmes or presentations relating to the sale of CAM products.

If you require work-space for carrying out administrative and practice-management tasks, then *hot-desking*, probably at a business centre, or working or holding presentations or meetings at *café or hotel premises* are options. However, these venues may present problems fulfilling the criteria mentioned above, especially with regard to the provision of a quiet, consistently available and confidential work-space or meeting place.

Commercial leasing of business premises can prove to be the most expensive option and involves matters which should be discussed with a Solicitor and a Chartered Surveyor. Identifying an appropriate trading location is vital and resources like Local Data Company can help with this (http://www.localdatacompany.com/). If you are planning to open a shop to sell products, a Health Centre or other treatment facility, it could be good business sense to promote a community spirit between your practice and neighbouring businesses, even when they are trading in competition with you, with the aim of swapping ideas and learning from each other. If neighbouring businesses are a success and bring more prospective customers to your area then this can benefit your practice too. Competition can be healthy.

Many businesses are opting to work from dedicated Business Centres and "Innovation Centres". These have the advantage of charging reasonable (sometimes subsidised) all-in rents or licence fees with flexible options for occupation, up-to-date facilities, car-parking availability and compliance with workplace legislation and regulations. This business environment could be particularly attractive to a Practitioner whether for the provision of treatment rooms or for providing facilities for the manufacture and sale of products.

Here are some examples:

http://www.innovationcentrehastings.com

http://www.regus.co.uk/

http://www.canterburyinnovationcentre.co.uk/

OTHER PRACTISING VENUES

Some businesses promote their products and services from other venues called *'Pop-up Businesses'* or *'Pop-up shops'*. An example of the former, in the context of general business, could be where a café business uses trading premises in the day when the same premises are used for a different business (e.g. for the running of a bar) during the evening. Where a business is concerned with selling a product which needs to be displayed to customers, a business owner could adopt the low-cost and low-risk option of testing the market by setting up a pop-up shop for a limited trial period, possibly only for a few hours or days. This could be in empty, appropriately located retail premises (after taking the advice of local estate agents) or in less traditional places such as a community hall. Venues of this kind could provide an excellent way to test a new product or to introduce and promote new health services to prospective clients.

You could also consider holding a *Pop-up Event* to promote your practice.

HEALTH CENTRE: PRACTISING IN OR OWNING

You may decide to practise in a Health Centre where you can enjoy the benefits of working in association with other Practitioners providing multi-disciplinary complementary therapies to clients. Some Health Centres include retail premises from which you could arrange to sell your CAM or Therapy products. As your practice develops and expands, it may be that you decide to start your own Health Centre in which case you will have the freedom to develop it as your business. Whether working in a Health Centre or owning one, you will find the following suggestions useful.

SUGGESTIONS FOR THE PRACTICE MANAGEMENT OF A HEALTH CENTRE:

Define the Practice Manager's relationship with:

- Practitioners
- Clients/Patients
- Local NHS General Practitioners, Consultants & Health Care Providers
- Local Hospitals & Clinics
- Social Care Sector
- Voluntary Sector

Create and keep updated a Health Centre Practitioner's Handbook:

The Centre's rules and requirements including assisting a client/ patient to choose a treatment and/or a Practitioner, the handling of incoming mail/messages (confidentiality) and the collection of fees.

Other matters to consider:

o *Legal relationship with Practitioners*: Employee/Self-employed? Implications

o *Licence to occupy to be granted to each Practitioner*: possible content/ requirement of independent legal advice

o *Disputes between Health Centre and Practitioner*: Need for a work-place mediation facility

o *Proposed Practitioner Board*: Membership/Constitution/ Parameters

o *Complaints procedure*: Internal and/or external; Involvement of Practitioner's professional Membership organisation

o *Vetting of Practitioner/Client Contract, Code of Care; Consent to treatment procedures; Parent or Guardian Consent to treatment procedures*

o *Vetting of Practitioner:* Membership registrations and professional Insurance (annually)

o *Professional Negligence Indemnity Insurance*: requirement for individual Practitioner and separate cover for Health Centre, the importance of "run-off" cover

o *Employer's Civil liability Certificate & Insurance and Public liability Insurance*: requirements

o *Membership* of, for example, the *Federation of Small Businesses (FSB)*: benefits

o *Membership of professional registers*: see Appendix at

the end of this book.

- ○ *The safeguarding of vulnerable groups*: Disclosure and barring service

- ○ *Legislation*: implications for some Practitioners

- ○ *Disability Discrimination Act:* need for premises assessment survey?

- ○ *Data Protection Act*: need to register and appoint a data controller? Cyber security protection?

- ○ *Practitioner's professional requirements* (if any) relating to statutory regulation or voluntary self-regulation

- ○ *Medical Health & Local Government Authorities*: Implications for Practitioners & Health Centre

- ○ *CAM research resources*: encourage Practitioners to make available for clients

- ○ *Health Centre Evidence-based CAM research guides* for display in Health Centre reception area: sources, content and format

- ○ *The creation of a CAM lending Library as a health centre resource* for the use of clients, practitioners and CAM students using the Centre

- ○ *Health Centre Newsletters* both internal (for Practitioners) and external (for existing and prospective clients)

- ○ *Arrange participation* in open days, trade fairs, expo exhibitions and CAM conferences

- ○ *Arrange Practitioner contribution to the marketing of their practice, the Health Centre & CAM generally:* local radio, television and other media outlets to include Practitioners giving interviews & presentations

○ *Arrange local competitions* (e.g.a *Picture of Health painting competition*) promoting Health Centre and its Practitioners

○ *Marketing*: website & social media content; Practitioner brochures – in a "house style"? Voucher scheme

○ *Provision of Training facilities*: meeting the increasing demand for Practitioner CPD Courses

○ *Place entries* in local Health Guides/Listings

○ *CAM product sales*: need for sales staff training/insurance

○ *Keep under review interaction and networking with local NHS & private health providers*

○ Promote the use of client *treatment records* and the use of *Treatment Evaluation Forms,* incorporating client-related *treatment outcome measures*

○ *Promotion of Integrated Healthcare practice ethics:* Practitioner mentoring; Promote integrated healthcare treatment plans

○ Create & distribute Health Centre reception information & therapy guides

○ *Review awareness of contra-indications between different types of treatments*: implement process for practitioner liaison & resolution of practitioner disputes

- Preparation for *local authority spot-check* inspections relating to *Health and Safety at Work* activities and records

- *Environmental Protection legislation*: annual waste declaration and compliance issues

- *Practitioners to complete accredited first-aid courses* (usually every three years) check that this has been done

- Encourage Practitioners (where appropriate) to obtain a *NHS National Independent Provider Organisation Code* and to register as a provider with private health insurance companies

- *Promote awareness of European Union proposals and Directives* relating to CAM

- *Liaise with relevant authorities* regarding approval of Health Centre for the practice of relevant treatments (e.g. for acupuncture)

- *Liaise with Social Services and GP Practices* with regard to referrals (e.g. for psychotherapy and counselling)

- *Generally encourage and advise Practitioners to adopt a business approach* to their CAM practice and to spend adequate time on as well as in their practice.

HOW TO PLAN YOUR PRACTICE

Read through the following website which provides information about how to plan your business. Don't be daunted by the extent and complexity of this information. It is intended to give you an overview.

www.moneydonut.co.uk/accounting/budgeting-and-cost-control/plan-and-budget-for-growth

And see also:

http://www.greatbusiness.gov.uk/

DEVELOP AND EXPAND YOUR PRACTICE: THE FUTURE

To become a larger business, for instance to facilitate an increase in the sale of your CAM or therapy retail products or to open a Health centre, you will almost certainly need to delegate to and empower trustworthy staff and support personnel. Read this section in conjunction with the sections on **EMPLOYING STAFF, OUTSOURCING, VIRTUAL ASSISTANT** and **FINDING PROFESSIONALS**.

The following government website will give you ideas about how to develop and expand your practice. When setting up your practice, you will need to make a decision about its structure. Will you operate as a *Sole Trader*, as a *Partner* in a *Partnership* or will you incorporate your business as a *private limited Company* or adopt some *other form* of business structure? As your business develops and expands, its structure may need to change.

http://www.gov.uk/browse/business/setting-up

Also explore the Government's "Business is Great" website:

http://www.greatbusiness.gov.uk/

If your practice's objective is to serve the community, you could set up a *Social Enterprise* or a *Community Interest Company*:

http://www.gov.uk/set-up-a-social-enterprise

If you are a student who would like to start a practice or work in one then investigate the website of the *National Association of College & University Entrepreneurs:* http://nacue.com/

RESEARCH YOUR COMPETITORS

Explore the websites of those practices that compete with yours. Use them to get ideas about how to operate and promote your practice and learn how to assess your competition.

Links to the websites of other practitioners can be found in the 'find a practitioner' sections of relevant membership organisations and regulators, examples of which are detailed in the Appendix at the end of this book.

With regard to the manufacture and sale of products, business information may be found on relevant trade association websites:

http://www.taforum.org/

or by searching for 'tailored selection links' at:

http://www.greatbusiness.gov.uk

Useful information may also be found on career-focused websites such as:

http://tinyurl.com/c9x9fwd (*National Careers Service*)

So, before you start your practice or develop a business sales initiative, take the time to undertake online investigation of other practices that provide the same or similar business models as those that you propose to offer, particularly those trading in your practice's market area and with whom you will be in competition.

FINDING CLIENTS FOR YOUR PRODUCTS AND SERVICES

Review information about how to research your market:

www.marketingdonut.co.uk/market-research/market-research

Before using a *research consultant* or *agency,* refer to the *Market Research Society's Buyer's Guide*:

http://www.theresearchbuyersguide.com/

EXPORTING SERVICES AND PRODUCTS: ENTERING OVERSEAS MARKETS

Many small businesses adopt a trading area in and around the locality of their main business address. This would be the case in relation to a shop or Health Centre engaged in local retail sales of products or with regard to a practice providing health services to a particular community. Other businesses promote their products or services within the wider United Kingdom.

There are others that grow their businesses and enhance their profits by exporting to overseas markets. Small businesses have the flexibility to adapt and to respond to exporting opportunities and should not be put off by the rules, regulations and challenges associated with exporting. There is a great deal of advice and support available, for instance from Government Departments, see below, and from independent trade organisations like the *British Exporters Association:* http://www.bexa.co.uk/ *(BEXA).*

As a prospective exporter of CAM or therapy products, you should, in particular, focus your research and planning on defining the extent of your commitment, resources, marketing (pricing and promotion) and sources of finance (refer to the BEXA's publication: *'Guide to Financing Exports'*). Using local knowledge (appointing local agents in the target country) and adjusting the policies and procedures of your business to accommodate diverse cultures and customs are also essential challenges that you need to plan for before exporting commences. As ever, professional advice should be sought from the outset, not least to ensure that you have the correct legal and export documentation in place (preferably subject to English law) together with appropriate insurance cover (for example to cover marine/transit and late payment by your customers).

UK Export Finance:

The UK government website can provide advice on insurance if this is not available from the private market. You will also need to prepare for other matters like customer credit checks, customs requirements, currency exposure and taxation issues, including 'Delivered Duty Paid'.

The Department for International Trade (website below) can appoint an *International Trade Advisor* to assist you with your research and to help you with finding your target market and prospective customers. The *Trade Access Programme* provides funding to attend trade shows and missions worldwide.

If you are selling products overseas, consider appointing and learning from an experienced and reputable *International Distributor (ID)* who should have the necessary local knowledge, language skills and contacts together with an established customer list. Before appointing, you should meet and run checks on a prospective ID who should always pay up-front and be prepared to agree (in a legal document) the extent of the resources, commitment, time and money that he or she will contribute to marketing your product.

You could approach your Bank and your local and national business support organisations (refer to the relevant sections of this book) for assistance and advice, which is also available from:

The Department for International Trade: www.exportingisgreat.gov.uk

Open to Export: http://opentoexport.com/

HMRC: https://www.gov.uk/starting-to-export

The Enterprise Europe Network: http://een.ec.europa.eu/

Refer, also, to the **FINDING PROFESSIONALS** section of this book. Help might also be available from your local Chamber of Commerce http://www.britishchambers.org.uk/

ADVERTISING: CREATING A CAMPAIGN

Why should your clients attend your practice or buy your products and services rather than those of your competitors?

As when using the other marketing tools referred to in this book, including your website, printed material and social media, creating an advertising campaign requires that you use the right advertising methods at the right time and in the right place. Advertising summer garden furniture in the middle of winter or placing an advertisement aimed at young people in a publication that is mainly read by the elderly, is likely to prove a waste of resources. You should decide upon your target market (local, national or overseas?) and then plan your advertising campaign according to what your prospective clients want.

Get feedback from your clients and seek their views and those of your colleagues and even those of other advertisers. In-depth analysis of client feedback is crucial. For instance, did they understand the pricing element of your advertisement? Did they approve of your sales methods, for example your use of cold-calling or social media or your choice of publication? Does your brand communicate the message you intend? Generally, why are your clients buying or not buying what you are selling? Would they have been encouraged to buy if the advertisement had included the offer of a free sample of your product or a treatment or consultation at a reduced or waived fee? For example, a Chiropractor might offer prospective clients "a 15 minute free spinal check".

You could instruct a member of the *Chartered Institute of Marketing:* http://www.cim.co.uk/Home.aspx to undertake market research and analysis on your behalf, including a *'SWOT* analysis of your practice's or product's strengths, weaknesses, opportunities and threats.

For website tools, consider exploring the services of *Google Ad Words:* http://adwords.google.com and making use of *Google Analytics:* http://www.google.com/analytics/

Generally, your campaign should plan for the long-term, as it may take a number of advertisements to communicate with your client. Assess how many product sales you will need to make or treatments you will need to give in order to recover the cost of your advertising campaign. Remember, aiming to create 'brand awareness' in the marketplace when you are a small business could be a mistake if your competitors are large and able to draw on extensive marketing budgets. In this case it would be better to focus on creating a good quality, properly targeted and cost-effective advertising campaign.

Design your advertisement to be short and concise. It is likely that it will only have a few seconds to make an impression on your prospective client.

ADVERTISING STANDARDS AUTHORITY LTD. (ASA)

Review the compliance criteria imposed by the ASA (www.asa.org.uk) and explore the **Advertising Certification** facility available at www.grcct.org

Refer to the **SOCIAL MEDIA**, **FINDING YOUR MARKET** and **MARKETING PLAN** sections of this book.

LOCAL BUSINESS SUPPORT: ASK FOR HELP

Ask for help from local business support organisations. For example, here is an organisation which offers support services to businesses based in the South East of England:

http://www.letsdobusinessgroup.co.uk/ and join your local branch of the British Chambers of Commerce

http://www.britishchambers.org.uk/

NATIONAL BUSINESS SUPPORT: HELP IS AVAILABLE

You need not be alone. Although, as a Practitioner, you will have the support of your professional membership organisation and your practice's regulator, you could also join a national organisation which provides general business support and benefit from sharing ideas and strategies with other business owners who may, in due course, even become clients of your practice or purchasers of your products.

The Federation of Small Businesses (annual membership fee payable) provides membership benefits:

http://www.fsb.org.uk/benefits

and support services, including a legal advice helpline, legal documentation and templates and insurance quotations.

You could also join an online business support club, like *Enterprise Nation* (www.enterprisenation.com/) or the *New Entrepreneurs Foundation* (www.newentrepreneursfoundation.co.uk/) and keep up to date with new developments and enjoy online networking.

Useful information is available from The *British Chambers of Commerce:* http://www.britishchambers.org.uk/ and may be found in the *SME Insider's* Newsletters: http://www.smeinsider.com/

If you have opened a shop or are planning to do so, the following website provides training and advice for independent shopkeepers:

http://www.savethehighstreet.org/

A practice which includes family members could present

challenges and advantages. It might be sensible for each member of the family to manage a different aspect of the business and provide different treatments or therapies. Such businesses can enable parents and their children who are in the practice together to learn from each other and to share practising values. Useful advice and support may available form the *Institute of Family Business*: http://www.ifb.org.uk/

Practitioners who wish to acquire a focused entrepreneurial attitude, for instance to attain business skills for use in the sale of their CAM and therapy retail products, could explore the 'free business accelerator for early stage and growing ventures' provided by *Entrepreneurial Spark*: http://www.entrepreneurial-spark.com/.

SOURCES OF FINANCE

This section will be of interest to Practitioners who require funds to start-up or develop their practice or implement or increase their CAM or therapy product range.

As well as discussing this with your bank manager or an independent financial adviser, you could explore online information about other sources of funding, for example:

http://www.gov.uk/business-finance-support-finder

If you are starting a business, or if your business is at an early stage, review the Government's *Start up loans scheme* which is a government funded scheme that provides advice, business loans and mentoring services:

http://www.startuploans.co.uk/ and http://www.letsstartup.co.uk/

Investigate *Crowdfunding* sites. These are an increasingly popular source of funding for small, medium and start-up businesses. *Crowdfunding* permits you to raise even a small amount of money from any number of investors. Put simply, this source of finance allows entrepreneurs to raise funding online by either selling some equity in their business (the equity share model) or by giving away rewards (the rewards based model), like selling a CAM product to the funder at a reduced sale price or by entitling the funder to learn about your business process. There is also a 'lending model' which does not offer equity or reward but which does entitle the funder to a return on their investment. In this way, your business also has an opportunity to acquire clients before it has even started. Examples are:

http://www.crowdcube.com/

http://www.seedrs.com/

The above and other crowdfunding sites have enabled many small and medium sized businesses, community organisations and charities to raise finance that they might otherwise have been unable to secure (http://bit.ly/1EQkooM). *The Crowdfunding Association* (http://www.ukcfa.org.uk/) was formed in 2012 and, amongst other things, aims to *'promote crowdfunding as a valuable and viable way for UK businesses, projects or ventures to raise funds'*.

It is vital that you fully research the form of crowdfunding that best suits your CAM products and services. You should personally engage with your prospective investor before you make your fundraising application, for instance by using video or other visual means that will permit the investor to 'look you in the eye' via their computer screen. Before you go online, you will need to have your comprehensive Business and Marketing Plans in place, which should contain the information that the investor wants to see, including information about your experience and the potential market share of your business proposal. A successful application and online pitch must motivate and engage with the investor if it is not to fail. Speak to as many successful applicants as you can and learn from their experience.

Although, possibly, a less-popular option for a Practitioner, you might also consider approaching your clients for funding, for instance to raise funds for product-development. *Customer-funding* can, for example, be by way of advance payment arrangements or subscription and does not require you to give up equity or pay loan interest. It is also a way of testing the potential of your product or services. If your client is not prepared to pay for them in advance, then it maybe that they would not buy them from you in any case. Once again, make your approach to the client as personal as possible. Avoid emails and write a handwritten letter and then follow this up with a telephone call. Your client needs to trust you as well as the product or services you will be providing.

Another form of capital raising is by way of *Peer to Peer Lending* websites. These websites match savers who are willing to lend with borrowers, who may be individuals or small businesses. Information and analysis is available from Which? (http://www.which.co.uk/).

Explore the lending requirements of *Business Angels* (https://www.ukbaa.org.uk) and be ready to give the prospective lender a clear explanation of what the loan is for and how he or she will get their money back together with a statement of your practice's profit and loss, turnover and overheads. Approach Business Angels who know about your type of practice and products and take references about them from other borrowers. You need to trust and, preferably, like each other.

If you are proposing to manufacture and sell your products on a large scale, you may be able to raise *inward investment* finance from a foreign investor who is prepared to invest in your business as a result of increasing globalisation. Such investors may be from the Middle East, Africa, Russia or China. Online information is available from Invest UK (http://www.investuk.com/) which claims to be the '*market leader in bringing foreign direct investment into unlisted UK companies*'. The Department for International Trade also supports inward investment projects (https://www.gov.uk/government/organisations/uk-trade-investment). If it is appropriate for your business, then you might want to think about networking and building relationships with foreign investors. Finally, it is important to keep in mind that investors will almost certainly want to have a clear exit strategy. They will want to know when they can expect to receive a financial return on the investment risk they are taking.

Other websites which may be of interest are:

The British Bank PLC (a development bank wholly owned by HM Government): http://british-business-bank.co.uk/

The National Association of Commercial Finance Brokers (NACFB): http://www.nacfb.org/

Independent and regulated Financial Advisers: https://www.unbiased.co.uk/

The ICAEW: http://www.icaew.com/en/about-icaew

Business Banking Insight: http://www.businessbankinginsight.co.uk/

Financial Conduct Authority: http://www.fca.org.uk/

PREPARE YOUR MARKETING PLAN

Research information about marketing your practice:

www.marketingdonut.co.uk/market-research/market-research

Apart from setting up your own business premises in the location where you want to practice there are other ways to bring your product or services to the marketplace. You could find a partner who is already established in a practice, although for this you would expect to sacrifice some control and financial return. You could enter the market by acquiring an existing practice, provided you had first secured the funding to do so and also properly and successfully completed the necessary checks, research and business planning.

One of the best ways to market your practice is to ask satisfied clients to recommend you to their friends and colleagues, so obtain feedback from your clients (www.surveymonkey.com) and respond swiftly to their needs. The use of social media, like Facebook and Twitter, is mentioned in the social media section of this book. Any information that you hold about your clients, sometimes referred to as a *client list* or *client database*, is likely to be of enormous use to your marketing plans. When and why did they buy from you and how can you keep in touch with them? Converting a past client into a repeat client may be achieved simply by maintaining contact, for instance by using relevant software (http//www.constantcontact.com) and see also http://www.aweber.com/index-trialzero.htm

Your clients need to know where to find you. Refer to the ADVERTISING and SOCIAL MEDIA sections of this book and *implement a joined-up marketing and advertising campaign* which could include the following means of communicating with your clients:

- An email newsletter to existing clients (refer to the WRITING ARTICLES & NEWSLETTERS section of this book);

- Exhibit at a Trade Fair or at a Business Event (see, for example, *Let's Do Business Group* exhibitions: http:// www.letsdobusiness.org/);

- Issue a press-release to publications relevant to your practice;

- Advertise in appropriate print publications, adding a QR code;

- Post on Facebook and Twitter;

- Post podcasts and upload videos about your products and services;

- Post Blogs in appropriate forums;

- Appear on local radio and television channels to talk about your practice and/or products;

- Produce a good quality practice brochure and other printed publicity material;

- Distribute flyers in a direct-mail campaign;

- Display advertising on billboards and posters;

- Attend networking events;

- Implement a sales-call process;

- Publish across multiple networks and social profiles

(http://sproutsocial.com/).

Seek *Endorsements* from organisations that also have dealings with your clients. You can then place these on your marketing material, online and offline, together with the endorser's logo, if permitted.

PRICING STRATEGIES: THE CHARGE FOR YOUR SERVICES AND THE PRICE OF YOUR PRODUCT

Investigate what your competitors are charging. The web-links in the Appendix will assist you with this. Review the following general business information about pricing strategies:

www.marketingdonut.co.uk/market-research/benchmarking/ choose-a-pricing-strategy

Here is a useful Blog view by William Levins which could assist you with pricing your product:

https://www.nuvonium.com/blog/view/how-to-price-your-product-for-retail-distributor-and-direct-to-consumer-sal

PARENT AND WOMEN PRACTITIONERS

The Federation of Small Businesses has published a report *Women in Enterprise: The Untapped Potential*:

Search at: http://www.fsb.org.uk/media-centre/publications/?q=women

If you are a mother, explore a source of networking links and useful information relevant to mothers who are also Practitioners:

http://www.mumpreneursnetworkingclub.co.uk/

http://www.workingmums.co.uk/

Mothers and women constitute a significant number of business owners who use the services of *Start-up Britain* (http://www.startupbritain.org) a government-backed campaign to encourage new businesses. See also https://shemeansbusiness.fb.com/

Your local *Family Information Service (FIS)* provides information about all services available to parents. Search the following link to get in touch with your FIS for details of childcare and early years provision in your area:

http://findyourfis.daycaretrust.org.uk/kb5/findyourfis/home.page

Further help and advice is available from the *Family and Childcare Trust*:

http://www.familyandchildcaretrust.org/

The charitable organisation *Gingerbread* provides advice and practical support for single parent families:

http://www.gingerbread.org.uk/

CHANGE OF CAREER AND NEW PRACTITIONERS OVER 50

If you are over 50 years of age and planning to start a practice, explore events and advice provided by *Enterprise Nation* through its *50 Plus: Events for people over 50 wanting to become their own boss* programme:

https://www.enterprisenation.com/50plus

If you are thinking of leaving your current job and *changing your career*, whether by choice or through necessity, you need to plan for the change.

Think carefully why you are making the change and what you will need to do to fully attain what you want to achieve in your new career. You need to be sure that you will continue to be satisfied with your choice of new career. What is your ambition and is it realistically achievable? Do you want to embark on a completely new career as a Practitioner or would you prefer a career related to your previous employment, which is likely to require less adjustment and re-training? You only need to change to the extent that it is necessary for you to be content with your new career, which may not mean that you have to completely reinvent yourself.

If you have a particular type of practice in mind, arrange to spend time with and talk to Practitioners so that you can assess its career problems as well as its rewards.

If you are a former member of the armed forces who is looking to start a practice, have a look at http://www.x-forces.com/ which is a service that provides funding support and advice for services-leavers, military spouses, veterans, and reservists who would like to start their own business.

FINDING PROFESSIONALS

It is prudent to take professional advice about your business early in the process. Leaving this until it is too late can prove to be an expensive mistake.

To find a Chartered Accountant in your area, search:

http://www.icaew.com/en/about-icaew/find-a-chartered-accountant

http://www.searchaccountant.co.uk

To find a lawyer, search:

http://tinyurl.com/bw5k33r : Solicitor

http://www.cilex.org.uk/ : Chartered Legal Executive

http://www.barcouncil.org.uk/using-a-barrister/public-access/: Barrister (Public Access).

Appoint a reputable Bank and Banker to administer your business bank account(s): https://www.ukfinance.org.uk/

It is important to keep your personal and business finances separate as this will avoid confusion and also assist you or your Chartered Accountant when the time comes for you to prepare and submit your end of year business accounts to HMRC.

Finding a professional adviser through personal recommendation is also a good starting point but always enquire first whether the person you intend to instruct is an expert in the type of advice you need.

VIRTUAL RECEPTION AND BUSINESS ADDRESS: FACILITIES

If your practice's business address and proposed trading area is based by the sea, then half of your target market area could be said to be "in the sea". In these circumstances and if it is your intention to sell your product outside your local area, you could consider acquiring a business address and virtual reception facilities situated further inland. Similarly, a rurally based business could, if desired, acquire a possibly more prestigious city-centre presence.

Regardless of where you are located, if you are working from home you might prefer to have a business address, business reception and answering service separate from your home address. If this is the case do some research about virtual-office facilities, including on the following websites:

http://www.receptionbureau.co.uk/

http://www.regus.co.uk

http://sussexbusinessbureau.co.uk

http://www.hbolsussex.co.uk

PRACTICE WEBSITE

Having a website will help to promote your practice and products.

An informative and well designed website is a very important marketing tool. If, at the outset, you are not able to afford a professionally built site, you could self-build a basic site using, for example:

Wix:	http://www.wix.com
Wordpress:	http://wordpress.com/
BaseKit:	www.basekit.com
Mr Site:	www.mrsite.com
Moonfruit:	www.moonfruit.com
1&1:	www.1and1.co.uk

Your business website is your world-wide shop window. It informs your clients about who and where you are and about what you do and when you do it. Keep it up to date with new, good quality content. Be prepared to spend an hour a day posting content and responding to clients enquiries. When you have generated sufficient income using the internet, you will have the option of outsourcing some of these activities to a social media professional.

Make sure that your website is mobile-user friendly: https://www.google.com/webmasters/tools/mobile-friendly/.

SEARCH ENGINE OPTIMISATION

Remember to maximise your search engine optimisation (SEO) so that your business website is noticed by users and search engines. There is no point in owning an excellent website which, nevertheless, fails to promote your practice and products simply because they are not being seen by prospective clients. This would be like owning a shop full of desirable stock which has the blinds drawn over its shop window. It is effectively closed for business. Research *Google's keyword search tool* and *Google Insights* to assess the relevance and effectiveness of your website's keywords.

For further information and website links, please refer to the Social Media section of this book.

YOUR PUBLIC PROFILE ON LINKEDIN

Create or expand your existing public profile on LinkedIn. Spend about 20 minutes a week updating your profile and strengthening your network and testimonials:

http://www.linkedin.com/

MARKETING AND PROMOTIONAL MATERIAL

For online purchase of print-copy marketing and promotional material and business cards you could contact 'Moo Print' or 'Vista Print':

http://uk.moo.com/

http://www.vistaprint.co.uk

INTELLECTUAL PROPERTY

You or your practice may own some form of Intellectual Property. This might be an artistic design, shape, technology or a brand of treatment process or product. For information about how to protect and exploit your intellectual property assets, review the following:

http://www.ipo.gov.uk/types.htm

http://www.gov.uk/browse/business/intellectual-property

If you are concerned about protecting your business idea, only discuss it with people you trust. Concern about confidentiality could be resolved by the completion of a non-disclosure agreement. For this, you should consult a lawyer.

DATA PROTECTION AND CYBER SECURITY

Your practice will almost certainly handle personal and health information about your clients in which case you may have a statutory legal obligation to protect such information under *Data Protection* legislation. For instance, you may require a *Data Protection Licence* (renewable annually):

http://www.ico.org.uk/

According to the *National Fraud & Cyber Crime Reporting Centre (ActionFraud)*:

'...With online crime becoming an increasing threat for business, new figures from Get Safe Online and Action Fraud show that from March 2015 - March 2016, a huge total of £1,079,447,765 was reported lost by businesses to online crime. This comes as Action Fraud saw a 22% increase from 30,475 in 2014 - 2015, to 37,070 crimes reported in the last year. On average, each police force in the UK recorded £19,626,323 in losses by businesses in their area. However, the true picture could be even higher, as these figures do not take into account the amount potentially lost by those who choose not to report online crime to the police...' (http://bit.ly/29jCJBW)

Read more about cyber security advice for small firms at:

https://www.gov.uk/government/news/small-firms-urged-to-take-steps-to-combat-cyber-crime

https://www.cyberaware.gov.uk and https://www.getsafeonline.org/

Your practice might be attacked through website hacking, malicious codes (trojans and viruses) and 'ransomware', which is a code that encrypts everything on the infected computer until the ransom is paid. Some very simple measures can assist with combatting these: choose secure passwords, keep software up-to-date, train yourself and staff to appreciate why security precautions are necessary and ask your information technology suppliers about the security of the services they provide to your business.

Helpful advice is also available from the *Information Commissioners Office* (http://www.ico.org.uk/) and the *Information Assurance Consortium (IASME)*, which is one of the *Cyber Essentials* accreditation bodies appointed by the UK Government (http://www.iasme.co.uk).

Review the guidance provided by The National Cyber Security Centre at www.ncsc.gov.uk

DISCLOSURE AND BARRING SERVICE

If your practice will be employing people or recruiting and hiring then certain types of jobs or voluntary work, especially where engaged in healthcare, may require a *Disclosure and Barring Service* check and certification (previously called a 'Criminal Records Bureau' check):

http://www.gov.uk/disclosure-barring-service-check

EMPLOYING STAFF

Many Practitioners practise alone as sole-practitioners. However, as their practice develops or as the sale of their products increases, it may become necessary for them to employ staff.

If you will be employing staff, take a look at the following guidance:

https://www.gov.uk/employing-staff

and review these *ACAS* guides:

http://www.acas.org.uk/index.aspx?articleid=4231

According to the Department for Business, Innovation and Skills (2014), which has been replaced by the Department of Business, Energy & Industrial Strategy, small and medium-sized businesses account for 59% of private sector employment and 48% of private sector turnover. Small businesses, those with less than 50 employees, alone account for 47% of private sector employment and 33% of private sector turnover.

As the owner of your business you need to communicate effectively with your employees. This can be assisted by keeping them informed (e.g. by holding reasonably frequent meetings) about business performance and matters that will affect them, taking an interest in what they do both at work and, if they think it appropriate, even outside work; where possible, avoid using emails and instead speak to them in person; give praise when it is due and ask them for their views; listen to what they have to say and consider their useful proposals; where appropriate, be prepared to change in response to what you learn.

It is advisable to take legal advice about your *employee's entitlements* both at the time they start to work for your business and during the course of their employment. It is good practice to keep your employment policies and procedures under review and to check that they continue to reflect the changing needs of your practice.

When recruiting an employee, consider using social media as a recruitment tool. Facebook, Twitter and YouTube can be used to advertise for new staff as well as to market your business and receive feedback. It is inexpensive, quick and transparent and it only requires an internet connection. LinkedIn (www.linkedin.com) provides the opportunity for you to view a candidate's linkedIn profile and, of course, gives the candidate the opportunity to view yours. This transparency facilitates a swift response from candidates to job advertisements, which can be especially helpful to a small business which often needs to fill a position at short notice. For a small annual fee, linkedIn also provides a specialist recruitment service.

Refer to the TAKING AN APPRENTICE section of this book.

Research and statistics relating to employment and skills in the UK:

www.gov.uk/government/organisations/uk-commission-for-employment-and-skills

The organisation *Investors in People* (http://www.investorsinpeople.com) states:

'We discovered that what really counts isn't strategy or technology or management structure. It's people. Study after study shows that an engaged workforce is critical to performance'

TAKING AN APPRENTICE

If you are thinking of taking an apprentice into your practice, have a look at:

http://www.greatbusiness.gov.uk/taking-on-an-apprentice/

http://www.apprenticeships.org.uk/

You would be required to provide work experience and specified skills together with a wage and holiday pay for the period of the apprenticeship, which can operate at 3 levels - intermediate, advanced or higher.

"Apprentices bring with them a wide range of benefits, from increased productivity and staff development to a fresh injection of ideas and a cost-effective way to build a talented workforce for the future. You could play a key role in a young person's development whilst growing your business." *

Graham Marley,

Chief Executive of Let's Do Business Group

(http://www.letsdobusinessgroup.co.uk/)

* From Sussex Business Times (SBT) Issue 384 (www.sussexbusinesstimes.co.uk).

OUTSOURCING

If you do not want to incur the cost or responsibility of employing staff or if you lack the skills and experience for specific tasks, you have the option of outsourcing those tasks to an external provider, for example in relation to IT, SEO, accountancy, recruitment and and other services.

If you do outsource, it is vital that you clearly define and agree, preferably in writing, the precise extent of the tasks outsourced.

Generally, you could outsource to other small businesses or to freelancers who you could instruct to act as your virtual workforce. This could be particularly useful for project assignments:

http://www.peopleperhour.com/?var1=1

Freelancer.co.uk

Upwork.com

For instance, bookkeeping for small businesses could be outsourced to a certified book keeper such as a Member of the *Institute of Certified Bookkeepers UK*:

http://www.bookkeepers.org.uk/

If you would like your CAM or therapy product to be made for you, investigate outsourcing their manufacture:

http://www.letsmakeithere.org/

http://makeitbritish.co.uk/

HIRE A VIRTUAL ASSISTANT

As a busy Practitioner involved in expanding your practice you could consider hiring a Virtual Assistant (VA) who you must be able to trust and who has the relevant niche skills and experience that you need, such as managing your website and social media, undertaking marketing, data entry or secretarial services. Some VAs work as freelancers for only a few hours a week whilst others work full-time or as one of a team of VAs who are able to offer a diverse range of skills. There are numerous online directories of Virtual Assistants operating in the UK, for example:

www.ukava.co.uk/

BUSINESS DIRECTORIES

When advertising your practice, make the most of local free online Business Directories. Here are some examples of business directories serving East Sussex in the South of England:

http://www.ieastsussex.co.uk

http://www.freeindex.co.uk/

http://www.sussexfind.co.uk

Nationally recognised UK business directories include:

http://trustedtraders.which.co.uk/

http://www.checkatrade.com/

http://www.checkaprofessional.com/

You could also, of course, use these directories to find a trade or service.

SOCIAL MEDIA: PROMOTE YOUR PRACTICE AND PRODUCTS

Social Media is an essential marketing tool. It's a good idea to use a combination of several types of media platforms. For instance, you could produce a short video about your practice's services and products and post it on YouTube which you could then link to your Facebook and Twitter accounts. Your 'followers' would then be able to "comment", "like" or "re-tweet" to all of their 'followers', thereby distributing information about your practice or products.

Information about Social Media may be found at: www.sproutsocial.com

With the world-wide proliferation of mobile phones, you might think it worthwhile building an *app,* preferably for a niche service or product. This will need to be marketed and updated if it is to have any chance of being successful (https:// developer.apple.com/).

While it is true that the internet will give a small business access to effective target-marketing, it is also true that the business will be competing with larger and better resourced brands. Internet marketing techniques are offered to the clients of providers like Captify (http://www.captify.co.uk/) which aims to help small businesses to advertise locally, nationally and globally.

Arguably, digital marketing is more effective when it is automated to create multiple advertisements backed by up-to-date technology and software that analyses responses from online social media campaigns. As with any marketing exercise, it is important that you know your clients and focus on providing the right content through the right social media networks. Apply the same approach as you would with face to face networking. Avoid being negative and using excessive sales-talk and jargon and do not spam. Take legal advice about the legal implications of using Social Media and, in particular, be careful not to violate confidentiality.

Training in digital marketing, including in the effective use of social media and search engine optimisation is available from providers like Jellyfish (www.jellyfish.co.uk).

Refer to the ADVERTISING section of this book.

WRITE ARTICLES AND E-NEWSLETTERS ABOUT YOUR PRACTICE AND PRODUCTS

Consider writing articles for professional journals relevant to your specialism, columns in newspapers and magazines and even appearing on local TV and radio broadcasts where an opportunity may arise to promote your treatments and products and, as an incidental outcome, the existence and location of your Practice. This can be a very successful way of raising your profile and that of your business.

Also consider producing a monthly or quarterly emailed newsletter, or e-letter, for distribution to those on your client database or client list and to other parties who have signed-up to receive it. A single page, possibly consisting of no more than 4 or 5 paragraphs outlining matters of interest, should be sufficient. The newsletter should also describe developments in your practice's services and products and provide a simple method of how to access more information about these. At the same time, review the media and Journals for items about your specialism and, of course, keep in touch with internet resources.

Useful websites are:

http://www.aweber.com/

http://mailchimp.com/

http://www.constantcontact.com

https://www.linkedin.com/

H. M. REVENUE AND CUSTOMS

You need to be aware of existing and anticipated H M Revenue & Customs (HMRC) policies that affect your practice. As I have mentioned before, it is recommended that you take the early advice of a Chartered Accountant. Prior to doing so, you might find it useful to review the following HMRC guidance about taxation and national insurance matters:

http://www.hmrc.gov.uk/webinars/index.htm

http://www.hmrc.gov.uk/selfemployed/

https://www.gov.uk/working-for-yourself

Free e-learning packages are available from HMRC to help you to understand what you need to know about tax, national insurance, expenses and record keeping, etc:

http://www.hmrc.gov.uk/courses/syob2/syob2/index.htm

Many local and national support organisations provide relevant training and business development courses.

TRAINING AND DEVELOPMENT

Practitioners will normally attend Continuing Professional Development (CPD) courses relevant to their specialism as required by their professional membership organisations and regulators.

Keeping up to date with your practise specialism, learning new skills and exploring new ways to deal with changes in your practising sector can improve your motivation and services and aid client satisfaction. Effective training can also reduce staff turnover and absenteeism.

A popular website for UK trainers which introduces a diverse selection of training topics is:

http://www.trainingzone.co.uk/

You could investigate general training and development programmes at:

https://www.nibusinessinfo.co.uk/node/14554

Free e-learning packages are available from HMRC to help you to understand what you need to know about tax, national insurance, expenses and record keeping, etc:

http://www.hmrc.gov.uk/courses/syob2/syob2/index.htm

Training in digital marketing, including the effective use of social media and search engine optimisation is available from providers like *Jellyfish*: www.jellyfish.co.uk.

For free trade magazine subscriptions and downloads of technical documents, research:

http://www.tradepub.com/ (Search: *Healthcare & Medical*)

Many local and national support organisations (refer to the relevant sections of this book) provide business development training.

INSURING YOUR PRACTICE, MAKING A *WILL* AND A *LASTING POWER OF ATTORNEY*

Insurance cover will almost certainly be essential for your business. In an increasingly litigious and challenging business environment, it is a sensible precaution to arrange an appropriate insurance policy to protect your practice. Such cover could include protection against claims of negligence (professional indemnity), infringement of intellectual property, loss of documents or data, cyber attacks, public and employers liability, losses due to critical illness and personal accident and damage to business premises and equipment, environmental liability, product liability, product recall, business interruption, travel, private medical and legal expenses. If you do not have an insurance company in mind, you could consult an Insurance Broker:

http://www.biba.org.uk/

As a responsible Practitioner, you should give thought to what would happen to your business, your colleagues, employees, partner(s) and clients and to members of your family in the event of your death or loss of mental capacity. You should take legal advice about making a *Will* and also a *Lasting Power of Attorney*.

FRANCHISING

Even if you are in the early stages of preparing to start your practice, you may want to explore the business format of franchising. It is possible that, in due course, you might decide to enfranchise the practice or product you have established. Alternatively, you may wish, from the outset, to join a reputable and sustainable franchise and run your practice using a franchisor's brand, support and training.

If you decide to purchase a franchise and become a franchisee remember that you will be working with a business model created and controlled by the franchisor. You need to be sure that the franchise is a successful business model with an established trading record. As always, thoroughly research and plan your venture and take professional advice.

Question the franchisor about the business model and speak to other franchisees asking, for instance, how long it took them to make a financial return and what training and support they received from the franchisor. Generally, make sure that you know what you are buying. Don't sign any documentation until after you have discussed it with an expert and taken legal advice. Enquire what will happen if things don't work out for you. Will any deposit you have paid to the franchisor be refundable? In what circumstances will you be in breach of contract?

You could visit the annual *British and International Franchise Exhibition*.

Useful information may be found at:

http://www.thebfa.org/

COMMUNICATING WITH YOUR CLIENT AND MANAGING YOUR PRACTICE

From a purely business perspective, the aim of your practice is to find clients and then to sell your practice services and products to them. In this context, there are two aspects of your business management which must be given a special mention:

1. Effective communication with your client and business contacts;

2. Efficient use of your time when managing your practice and promoting the sale of your products.

In the following 2 sections of this book, I make suggestions about how you might achieve these by pursuing activities to promote yourself and your practice, and by adopting administrative procedures both for that purpose and in order to maximise the sale of your products.

I do not deal with the delivery and practice-management of treatments or therapies as these are matters of professional skill and ethics upon which a Practitioner should exercise their professional judgement and receive guidance from his or her membership organisation and regulator.

EFFECTIVE COMMUNICATION

- Be available in person or by telephone to speak to your clients and do your best to limit the use of email, text and voicemail.

- Ensure that your phone and business cards are easily accessible.

- Consider using a separate mobile for your business.

- If a client or business contact is not available, then ask their assistant or 'gatekeeper' to book or diarise a time for you to call again (preferably not later than the next day). In this way, your client or contact can arrange to be available and should feel obligated to receive your next approach.

- With regard to any 'follow-up' contact, aim to telephone rather than email or text and then, if appropriate, immediately confirm your conversation in writing.

- Use emails to confirm, rather than to initiate, projects and contact with your client.

- Arrange 'face-to-face' meetings and adopt a personal approach whenever possible.

- Make a note of the date, time and the content of a telephone call, conversation or meeting on your your file, including a record of the time you have spent.

- Use your diary effectively. Remember to agree a follow-up appointment (date, time & venue) at the end of the first meeting and further meetings, which then confirm in writing. You may find it useful to keep a print diary in addition to an online version.

- Show interest in what your clients and contacts have to say.

- Prepare in advance of a meeting, telephone call or networking event an *'Elevator Pitch'* (about 40/50 words) which simply, briefly and effectively describes your practice and products and what you aim to achieve. Preparation will enable you to be more fluent and to make the maximum use of the limited time you will have to introduce yourself and to engage the interest of a prospective client or contact. It is also essential to have a few words ready when you are, maybe unexpectedly, called upon to address a group, for instance at a business networking breakfast or at a Chamber of Commerce meeting.

- Keep your client informed about how you are progressing with a project, for instance in relation to the manufacture, sale and delivery of your product. Email them weekly with a brief progress report, even if it consists of only a few lines of information. Use and regularly update a whiteboard in your work-place as technology has been known to fail, even if only temporarily. Continually action plan and review the progress of projects and product sales.

- Never tell a client or contact that you have done something when you haven't, even if it is the next thing you plan to deal with. There is always the danger that you will be distracted and forget to complete the task, with the result that you may, eventually, have to explain your error when you might lose the trust and respect of your client and even endanger the project's outcome.

- Generally, when estimating, it is better to slightly over-estimate than to under-estimate, whether in relation to time or money.

- Think of ways to encourage your client to recommend your business. Remember that your client database or client list is your best marketing tool. Ultimately, you want your client to be so enthusiastic and interested about your product or services that they will want to recommend them and you to everyone.

If necessary, you could obtain advice from the public relations and communications industry: http://www.prca.org.uk/

THE USE OF YOUR TIME : TIME MANAGEMENT

Many Practitioners practise as a sole practitioner, either alone or in association with other Practitioners in a Health Centre. Others deliver their services on a voluntary basis at hospices, within the care sector or as "support services" for the NHS.

Although Practitioners may be very competent at planning the delivery of treatments and therapies, some find it difficult to allocate sufficient time to manage their practice's administrative tasks. This can result in serious problems for example with the collection of fees, cash-flow, product manufacture and delivery, people-management, business logistics and accountancy matters. Some of the following suggestions will be of particular relevance to Practitioners engaged in selling products as this is a commercial activity requiring a 'corporate' approach.

When you start a project, make a written scheme of action dates (use your office whiteboard) and put them in your diary and on your client's file. As you progress, monitor action dates and be prepared to amend them, always remembering to keep your client well informed of anticipated delays and problems. Always work to a project completion date.

If necessary, you may need to dedicate a whole day, or more, to performing administrative matters, in which case plan ahead and allocate time for the day's tasks. Here (as only an example) is a daily work-scheme. This should be interpreted flexibly as you will, of course, need to adapt it to reflect your business activity and work-style.

7.30 to 9.00
attend a business networking breakfast (e.g. Chamber of

Commerce or Federation of Small Businesses)

09.00 to 09.30

plan your business activities for the day. Review your diary. What do you need to work on today? Which clients and contacts do you need to liaise with today? How? Why? Do you need to revise action dates and plans? Do you need professional advice or other help and support?

09.30 to 10.15

arrange (by telephone rather than email) 'face to face' meetings with clients, contacts and assistants;

10.15 to 10.30

take a break;

10.30 to 11.30

work on business plans and projects. Deal with business emails and business networking (delay dealing with personal matters until a leisure break or until the end of the working day);

11.30 to 13.00

attend meetings and work on business plans and projects;

13.00 to 14.00

leisure time or business lunch;

14.00 to 17.30

work on business plans and projects;

17.30 to 18.00

deal with business emails and business networking;

18.00

finish working on your business, deal with personal emails and focus on social, domestic and leisure activities.

* * * * *

Set up an email auto-responder and a voicemail confirming when you intend to reply to incoming emails and calls. This will appear efficient and professional to your clients and contacts who will prefer to know when they might expect to hear from you. It will also avoid the need for 'fire-fighting' and of being distracted by non-income producing activities. You may need to liaise with customers or contacts whilst working on projects but, when doing this, use your landline or mobile rather than email as this will usually save time.

Always answer your landline and mobile rather than leave it to divert to voicemail, unless you are giving a treatment or therapy, are in a meeting or necessarily unavailable or if it is not safe to do so (as when driving). The incoming call could be your most important existing or prospective client who may need you urgently and who may not be prepared to call again. By failing to take the call, you may miss a vital business opportunity.

Be prepared to make phone calls, particularly when arranging meetings. This should not be confused with 'cold-calling', which is often unproductive and, unless preferred, some business owners feel should be avoided. Making telephone calls is an essential part of running your business. Clients and contacts may want to hear a voice and be given the opportunity to assess the person who is or will be working on their behalf. For the same reason, it is important to adopt a personal approach and to agree to attend 'face to face' meetings.

Business meetings should take place at a business venue (preferably at a business premises, business centre or similar venue) or, if necessary, at a quiet and discreet public place such as an hotel, café or restaurant where confidentiality can be maintained. You should only agree to attend at a client's home if you are sure that this is appropriate, safe and professional.

Focus on completing one task before moving on to another.

Do not procrastinate. Deal with a matter rather than avoid it. Work to a sensible action plan and do not allow yourself to become overwhelmed.

Be careful not to overlook errors in process. For instance:

1. Is your profile on linkedIn (http://www.linkedin.com) and also the information posted on your website up to date?

2. Have you followed up prospective clients and those with whom you have previously been in contact? How long ago were they in touch? Have you forgotten someone?

3. How often do you need to revisit and reactivate your former clients and contacts? Have you 'saved' and 'backed-up' information for future action and implemented cyber crime protection?

4. Are you keeping to time limits, particularly with regard to regular invoicing and the action planning of projects?

5. Do you need to up-date your business documentation? Do your client Credit Terms or Terms & Conditions of Practice need revising?

6. Do you need to take professional advice, liaise with your bank or seek other support?

Prepare a matrix of all of your clients' names, contact details and project action dates, together with the dates for submission and payment of invoices. Keep an overview of the cash flow status and progress of your practice. Remember, cash flow is the lifeblood of any business.

Allocate time to prepare and send out invoices and interim invoices for payment. Consider collecting invoices by direct debit or by making use of card payment solutions. Also, your client may be prepared to pay by instalments or to make a deposit on a large invoice.

Allocate time to pay bills and to balance bank accounts and avoid paying extra bank charges and interest on debit balances.

Regularly review and update your Business Plan and Marketing Plan remembering to amend the figures in your Business Plan's financial pages, especially your Cash Flow Forecast. Review and update your cyber security.

Allocate time and funds for networking events, business conferences, trade fairs, training and continuing professional development courses. Join trade and business support organisations. To exploit international markets, for example at a trade fair, seek the advice and support of a Department for International Trade Export Adviser (www.exportingisgreat.gov.uk). Refer to the *Exporting: Entering Overseas Markets* section of this book.

Networking will expand your contacts and provide you with new ideas, so speak to as many people as you can and remember to make a note of their details (collect their business cards) so that you can follow up your new contacts, preferably the same or next day. Networking is a two-way process, so the more interested you are in the people you meet the more they are likely to reciprocate. If appropriate, make use of your *Elevator Pitch* to briefly explain your practice and products.

Be prepared to 'pitch' your business to prospective clients. Adequate preparation and subject research is vital, both to improve the content of your pitch and the confidence of your presentation. Although knowledge of your specialism forms the basis of your presentation, it is important that you have an assured demeanour and that you present a clear message. Beware of relying too heavily on *PowerPoint*, which has been described as 'computerised anaesthetic'. If you want to add a video or audio to your presentation (or to a document) take a look at: www.slidepresenter.com.

If necessary, consider training with a voice or business coach to enhance the quality of your delivery. Making a presentation may also provide an excellent opportunity to build business relationships, even when the presentation is not successful.

Get to know a prospective client before you make the pitch, perhaps by speaking to them on the telephone, if necessary on the pretext of discussing some relevant issues. Remember to follow-up your pitch, preferably the following day. Does your client have any questions? Would they like to have a meeting to discuss details? If your pitch was not successful, ask them if they would be prepared to give you some feedback? Learn from your client's feedback (https://www.surveymonkey.com/) and adjust your business policies and management procedures accordingly.

WRITE A BUSINESS PLAN FOR YOUR PRACTICE OR PRODUCT

You will have a much better chance of achieving your business goals if you first write them down. Make your business plan specific, realistic, achievable and measurable.

Having considered the information and resources referred to in this book, write or, if you already have one, update your Business Plan including the important financial pages.

A business plan is only a plan. Once prepared, it will need constant review and updating to reflect the changing nature of the market place and your business objectives and opportunities.

It may be used to check the progress of your business and to present to your professional advisers and business bankers when seeking their advice and support. For business plan advice and templates you could approach your Bank Manager and also research the following:

www.gov.uk/write-business-plan

www.greatbusiness.gov.uk/six-lessons

MENTORING

To assist you with your business plan (but not with writing it) and if you feel that you need help with the running of your practice, consider seeking the suggestions of a mentor. Mentoring has been described as *'An ear to listen, a brain to pick and a push in the right direction'.* It can make an enormous difference to the success of a new or even an established business. According to *The Federation of Small Businesses*, research has found that 70 per cent of small businesses which received mentoring survived for 5 years or more. This is double the rate compared with non-mentored entrepreneurs.

Ideally, your mentor will be from the same health sector and hold the same or similar specialism as your practice and will be someone that you feel will motivate you, with whom you can share ideas and plans and who will understand the challenges that your practice presents. Choose a mentor with whom you feel comfortable and who has the professional skills necessary to meet the needs of your business and, if possible, who will also be able to provide you with useful contacts.

Further information about mentoring may be found at:

http://www.greatbusiness.gov.uk/?s=Mentoring

http://www.mentorsme.co.uk/

http://www.horsesmouth.co.uk/ (Search: *business enterprise mentors*)

CONCLUSION

It is important to remember that your objective is to enjoy working in your own Practice.

Aim to complete treatments and practice-management tasks effectively and efficiently within a structured and properly time-managed working day.

Protect your leisure time and promote a healthy work-life balance. Try to avoid working at the weekend and, if you do, take equivalent time off during the week. Refer to the research carried out by the *Federation of Small Businesses*:

http://www.fsb.org.uk/policy/assets/work-life%20balance.pdf

Ultimately, the success of your practice and the sale of your products will be driven by your knowledge, personality and stamina.

I conclude with the following 'Top Tips' which apply to any business and which I reproduce with the kind permission of *First Voice,* the magazine of the *Federation of Small Businesses*:

1. *Know what you need to achieve and set yourself targets;*

2. *Have a plan and analyse what works well and how you can build on success to realise goals;*

3. *Do your research before meetings and ask the prospect appropriate open questions to help identify their needs;*

4. *Demonstrate the benefits of the product and how these will dovetail with the customer's needs;*

5. *Have self-belief, self-discipline and self-motivation and*

the sales will follow and have fun;

6. *Build rapport as people DO buy from people;*

7. *Build integrity and develop solid trust;*

8. *Deliver what you promise and, where you can, exceed expectations. Be remembered for the right reasons;*

9. *Try different tactics to reach targets and be creative;*

10. *Continuously build your knowledge and network of people to help you to reach your targets;*

11. *Call on your colleagues and contacts for mutual support as we all have 'off days';*

12. *Keep the prospect pot topped up and don't put all your eggs in one basket;*

13. *Don't forget to ask for the business;*

14. *Remember, 'givers gain' if you help someone, they are likely to want to help and do business with you.*

I hope that you have found this book useful. I wish you every success with your practice and with the sale of your products.

CHECKLIST

For Health Therapists and Practitioners of Complementary and Alternative Medicine:

- Will I remain committed to my practice and manage it as a business?

- Who will be my clients?

- Who will be my competitors?

- Having researched a market, should I target a 'Niche' market?

- Should I export my (therapy or CAM) product overseas?

- Is my product or service appropriately priced?

- Should I be advertising?

- Decide upon a business structure for my practice

- Nominate a practice address

- Do I need a 'Virtual Reception and Business Address' facility?

- Practising venues?

- Identify available local and national business support and mentoring services

- Does my business require financial support and, if so, what sources of finance are available?

- Appoint professional advisers

- Appoint a bank & open business bank account(s)

- Set up a website for my practice and maximise its

Search Engine Optimisation

- Create or expand and regularly update my linkedin profile

- Prepare printed marketing & promotional material

- Will my business own Intellectual Property and, if so, does it need legal protection?

- Identify my Data Protection responsibilities and implement Cyber Security protection

- Identify my Disclosure & Barring Service responsibilities

- Identify my responsibilities with regard to employing staff, freelancers or taking an apprentice

- Do I need the support of a Virtual Assistant?

- Do I need the help of others through outsourcing?

- Does my practice need to be listed in business or professional Directories?

- Should I belong to a trade association (product sales) or a professional organisation (services)?

- Does my practice need to be registered for legal or regulation purposes?

- Promote myself and my practice, including through:

- Use of social media

- Publishing articles in newspapers, magazines & trade or professional journals

- Local TV & Radio broadcasting

- By publishing monthly online e-newsletters to clients & interested parties

- Assess my business and personal status at HM Revenue & Customs

- Identify my personal and staff Training & Development needs

- Implement appropriate Insurance cover and make a Will and a Lasting Power of Attorney

- Create processes for effectively & efficiently communicating with my clients and contacts

- Implement time-management systems

- Remember to maintain a work-life balance

- Keep my Business Plan & Financial Pages up to date.

APPENDIX

Information for Health Therapists and Practitioners of Complementary and Alternative Medicine (CAM)

Please scroll down this page to find online links to the following:

- CAM articles by *Richard Eaton*

- Links to *Positive Health Online* and also to *The Alliance for Natural Health International*

- CAM organisations accredited by *The Professional Standards Authority*

- CAM research relating to a medical condition: *Cancer & Palliative Care*

- Research relating to a CAM treatment: *Homeopathy*

- General CAM Research resources

- CAM *Practitioner Organisations*

CAM ARTICLES BY RICHARD EATON

Details of Author

Published by *PositiveHealth Online* www.positivehealth.com

- Your CAM Practice and the Advertising Standards Authority – Time to take action a print version of this article is also available in Homeopathy in Practice Journal (Winter/Spring 2016) and in Journal of The Chartered Institute of Legal Executives (Parts 1 & 2: July/August 2016);

- Practitioners must state the case for complementary and

alternative medicine
including CAM research with a focus on *REIKI* also available in print, with a focus on *HOMEOPATHY* in: Homeopathy in Practice Journal (Autumn 2011);

- Complementary Medicine – Prepare for the Future;

- Complementary Medicine and the Voluntary Sector;

- Is choice of Healthcare a Human right? a print version of this article is also available in : Homeopathy in Practice Journal (Spring/Summer 2014) and in The Journal of The Chartered Institute of Legal Executives (CILEX): www.cilexjournal.org.uk/magazine

TO RECEIVE FREE Newsletters relating to Complementary and Alternative Medicine and for the Positive Health Research Archive REGISTER WITH Positive Health Online UK

REGISTER WITH www.anhinternational.org to receive information and Newsletters from The Alliance for Natural Health International

CAM ORGANISATIONS ACCREDITED by the *Professional Standards Authority*:

www.professionalstandards.org.uk/

CAM RESEARCH RELATING TO A MEDICAL CONDITION:
CANCER & PALLIATIVE CARE

'...The provision of complementary therapies is demanded by patients hence the services provided. Approximately 40% of breast and prostate patients use complementary therapies and 20% of patients with other cancers. The evidence and audits are very patient-centred and almost always supportive of the service and what it has to offer.

Complementary therapies are provided for patients, service users, carers and family members in almost every cancer and palliative care service in the country. Some of the most renowned cancer and palliative centres such as the Royal Marsden NHS Foundation Trust, Guy's and St Thomas's NHS Foundation Trust, St George's University Hospital NHS Foundation Trust, the Christie NHS Foundation Trust and a wide range of hospices and Macmillan cancer centres provide complementary therapies as an integral part of their supportive and palliative care services...'

Complementary & Natural Healthcare Council: February 2016.

www.cancerresearchuk.org/complementary-and-alternative-therapy-research

www.cancerresearchuk.org/complementary-therapy-organisations

www.cancerresearchuk.org/information-on-the-web

www.cancer.gov/about-cancer/treatment/cam

www.uclh.nhs.uk/OurServices/

www.positivehealth.com (search: *cancer articles* and *cancer research*)

The following links are only available in the e-book version of this book:

www.positivehealth.com/article/cancer/

www.positivehealth.com/article/cancer/cancer-target-cellular-respiration

www.positivehealth.com/article/cancer-diagnostic-tests

www.positivehealth.com/article/massage/

www.positivehealth.com/article/toxic chemo

www.positivehealth.com/new-cancer-fungus-theory

www.positivehealth.com/cancer/mistletoe-therapy-and-hyperthermia

www.positivehealth.com/article/cancer/deuterium-depletion

www.positivehealth.com/article/promising-cancer-treatments

www.positivehealth.com/article/streamlining-cancer-treatments

www.canceroptions.co.uk/

www.positivehealth.com/cancer/treatment-options

www.drsgoodman.com/book/nutrition-and-cancer

Resveratrol research papers:

https://www.ncbi.nlm.nih.gov/pubmed/28596842

https://www.ncbi.nlm.nih.gov/pubmed/20716633

https://www.ncbi.nlm.nih.gov/pubmed/11279601

https://www.ncbi.nlm.nih.gov/pubmed/26758628?log$=activity

Research and Information Initiatives:
PubMed: US National Library of Medicine, National Institutes of Health:
https://www.ncbi.nlm.nih.gov/pubmed/ (search "Cancer")
American Journal of Cancer Research:
https://www.ncbi.nlm.nih.gov/pmc/journals/1608/
Cochrane Library:
http://www.cochranelibrary.com/ (search "cancer")

www.homeopathy-ecch.org (Search: *cancer*)

Macmillan Cancer Support:

be.macmillan.org.uk/be/cancer-and-complementary-therapies

or a CD audio-book:

http://be.macmillan.org.uk/be/p-18885;

for information by Cancer type:

publications.macmillan.org.uk/

Cancer Research UK individual CAM therapies:

www.cancerresearchuk.org/about-cancer/

(Search: *complementary and alternative therapies*)

Cancer Research UK-research into Reiki for people with cancer:

www.cancerresearchuk.org/about-cancer/ (Search: *Reiki*)

Memorial Sloan Kettering Cancer Center:

www.mskcc.org/cancer-care/diagnosis-treatment

(Search: *Herbs,botanicals & other products*)

PubMed articles & clinical trials:

www.ncbi.nlm.nih.gov/pubmed

The Christie NHS Foundation Trust:

http://www.christie.nhs.uk/ ("Services: Complementary Therapy")

The Royal Marsden Hospital:

www.royalmarsden.nhs.uk/your-care/supportive-therapies

Support Organisations:

Marie Curie Cancer Care:

www.mariecurie.org.uk/

Macmillan Cancer Support:

www.macmillan.org.uk and see above

Penny Brohn UK:

www.pennybrohn.org.uk/

My Cancer treatment (NHS):

www.mycancertreatment.nhs.uk/

RESEARCH RELATING TO A CAM TREATMENT:

HOMEOPATHY

Faculty of Homeopathy:

http://facultyofhomeopathy.org/research/

Swiss Government Report:

anhinternational.org/2012/05/09/

Homeopathy Research Institute:

https://www.hri-research.org/

Homeopathy Research Institute clinical outcome research database:

www.hri-research.org/resources/research-databases/

The Society of Homeopaths:

http://www.homeopathy-soh.org/

The European Committee for Homeopathy:

http://www.homeopathyeurope.org/

International Council for Homeopathy:

http://www.homeopathy-ich.org/ich.html

CAM-quest database (click on the 'Therapies' quick-search box and select 'Homeopathy'): www.cam-quest.org

European Central Council of Homeopaths:

http://www.homeopathy-ecch.org/

British Homeopathic Association:

www.britishhomeopathic.org

HomBRex Database:

www.carstens-stiftung.de (search HomBRex Database)

The Alliance of Registered Homeopaths:

http://www.a-r-h.org/

Use of Homeopathy in Veterinary Medicine:

www.homeopathicvet.org/

British Homeopathic Dental Association:

http://www.bhda.co.uk/

The Homeopathic Medical Association:

www.the-hma.org

NHS Choices:

www.nhs.uk/Conditions/homeopathy/

Find a Homeopath:

http://www.findahomeopath.org/

N B The following links are only available in the e-book version of this book:

A research paper:

www.biomedcentral.com/

Article (Cancer):

http://www.positivehealth.com/article/cancer/

Establishing a scientific foundation in homeopathy (Constitutional prescribing):

www.a-r-h.org/wp-content/

Adaptive network nanomedicine: www.ncbi.nlm.nih.gov/

pubmed

GENERAL CAM RESEARCH RESOURCES

CAM-quest database:
http://www.carstens-stiftung.de/service/datenbanken
and see: www.cam-quest.org

Cancer Research UK:
www.cancerresearchuk.org/about-cancer/
and www.cancerresearchuk.org/complementary-alternative/

World Health Organisation:
"Traditional Medicine Strategy 2014-2023"
CAMbrella a pan-european research network for CAM:
http://www.cambrella.eu/home.php?il=8&l=deu

Norway's National research Center in CAM:
http://nafkam-camregulation.uit.no/

CAM for Cancer:
http://www.cam-cancer.org/
http://content.karger.com/

CamDoc Alliance:
http://camdoc.eu

CAMLIS: library information service
http://www.uclh.nhs.uk/ourservices/ourhospitals/rlhim/pages/
camlis.aspx

The Royal London Hospital for Integrated Medicine:
http://www.uclh.nhs.uk/ourservices/ourhospitals/rlhim/pages/
camlis.aspx

Pubmed: www.ncbi.nlm.nih.gov/pubmed

Cochrane Complementary Medicine:
cam.cochrane.org

The Research Council for Complementary Medicine:
www.rccm.org.uk

Bandolier:
www.bandolier.org.uk (Search: *complementary medicine*)

Positive Health Magazine (PH Online):
www.positivehealth.com

The University of Southampton – Complementary and
Integrated Medicine Research Unit
http://www.southampton.ac.uk/camresearchgroup

Camcomm:
www.camcomm.dk

The College of Medicine:
http://www.collegeofmedicine.org.uk/
www.collegeofmedicine.org.uk/complementary-medicine-blog

NHS Evidence – complementary and alternative medicine:

www.rccm.org.uk/node/11

NHS Conditions and Treatments:
www.nhs.uk/pages/home.aspx (search Complementary and Alternative Medicine)

International Society for Complementary Medicine Research:
www.iscmr.org

IN-CAM:
www.outcomesdatabase.org

Informed Health Online:
www.informedhealthonline.org

US National Library of Medicine:
www.nlm.nih.gov

National Center for Complementary and Integrative Health:
www.nccam.nih.gov

Samueli Institute:
www.samueliinstitute.org

University of Westminster CAM Degree Courses:
http://www.westminster.ac.uk/courses/subjects/complementary-medicine

Cochrane Evidence and Library:
www.cochrane.org/evidence (Search: *complementary medicine*)

European Federation for Complementary and Alternative Medicine:
http://www.efcam.eu/

Royal London Hospital for Integrated Medicine – Education Courses for statutory registered healthcare professionals:
www.uclh.nhs.uk/OurServices/

National Institute for Health & Care Excellence *(NICE)*:
www.evidence.nhs.uk/
www.patient.co.uk/doctor/complementary-and-alternative-medicine

British Medical Journal Clinical Evidence Review:
clinicalevidence.bmj.com/
or Google search Clinical Evidence efficacy categorisations

British Medical Journal (BMJ):
www.bmj.com/specialties/

Family Practice Oxford University Press Journals:
https://academic.oup.com/journals/ (search complementary medicine)

For information about REIKI research, treatments and training, refer to: www.marioneaton.co.uk (click on *Reiki Research* in the banner)
and see also
www.reikiinmedicine.org/medical-papers/

Cancer Research UK-research into Reiki for people with cancer:
www.cancerresearchuk.org/

For details of Reiki Training Courses
http://www.marioneaton.co.uk

CAM Reading List:
www.cancerresearchuk.org/

Complementary Therapies in Medicine Journal:
www.complementarytherapiesinmedicine.com/

Traditional, Complementary & Integrative Medicine –
an International Reader:

DISCERN Quality criteria for consumer health information:
http://www.discern.org.uk/

Yoga:
www.ncbi.nlm.nih.gov/pubmed/22041945

SOME CAM PRACTITIONER ORGANISATIONS

Complementary & Natural Healthcare Council:
http://www.cnhc.org.uk/

The General Regulatory Council for Complementary Therapies:
http://www.grcct.org/

Freedom4health:
http://freedom4health.com/about-us/

Complementary Medical Association:
www.the-cma.org.uk

British Complementary Medicine Association:
http://www.bcma.co.uk/

British Holistic Medical Association:
http://www.bhma.org/

Institute for Complementary and Natural Medicine:
http://icnm.org.uk/

Federation of Holistic Therapists:
http://www.fht.org.uk/

National Institute of Medical Herbalists:
http://www.nimh.org.uk/

British Association of Applied Nutrition and Nutritional Therapy:
http://bant.org.uk/

British Acupuncture Council:
http://www.acupuncture.org.uk/

British Medical Acupuncture Council:
http://www.medical-acupuncture.co.uk/

British Association of Art Therapists:
http://www.baat.org/

Association of Reflexologists:

http://www.aor.org.uk/

British Wheel of Yoga:
http://www.bwy.org.uk/

International Federation of Aromatherapists:
www.ifaroma.org/us/home/

International Federation of Professional Aromatherapists:
http://www.ifparoma.org/

General list with addresses:

Positive Health Online Magazine
www.positivehealth.com

Integrative Medicine (USA, Europe, Australia, China & India):
http://exploreim.ucla.edu/references/professional-associations/

British Association for Counselling and Psychotherapy:
www.bacp.co.uk

For homeopathy organisations see *ante*:
RESEARCH RELATING TO A CAM TREATMENT:
HOMEOPATHY

LEGAL NOTICE:

This Appendix provides information not medical advice. You should consult your medical practitioner if you have any symptoms of illness or concerns about treatment. Do not cease a prescribed conventional treatment without consulting your doctor. Tell all the practitioners you are working with, conventional or complementary, about any medicines, remedies, herbs or supplements you are taking or considering using.

No assurance, guarantee or promise is given with regard to the correctness, accuracy, up-to-date status or completeness of the information and websites for which there is no endorsement. Readers are strongly advised to discuss the information with their General Medical Practitioner, Medical Consultant and Healthcare Professional. No liability is accepted for any damage or loss caused to anyone who relies on the information and websites.

REVIEWS

This book is based on the first book in the series titled *Owning a Business: Things you need to Know*, for which the following reviews were kindly given: bit.ly/1REoab

"It is one of THE most comprehensive 'how to' and 'go to' start up business books I have ever read. Not just start up in fact, many small business owners will find information in there that will undoubtedly be useful in growing their businesses. 'Owning a Business' has a considerable amount of up-to-date information crammed into this deceptively slim volume, for example: information about crowd funding which the reader might not have considered. In summary: there is nothing left out, a very valuable purchase and must read. Buy it and TAKE ACTION!"
JENNIFER LINDLEY
Business Coach & Owner: Powerful People Performance

"The most relevant business start up and ownership book I have seen. In a few pages it reminds the reader of essential points and provides links to best practice. An excellent work. One to read before you start and to keep on the shelf for future reference."
CLIVE MARSH, Author
Financial Management for Non-Financial Managers: Kogan Page
Business and Financial Models: Kogan Page

"This was an excellent read with good clear advice for a business owner setting up and establishing a business. In addition, the information given is so comprehensive that it could also form part of a Bank Manager's toolkit when dealing with commercial customers."
NIGEL BISHOP, Senior Business Consultant
uk.linkedin.com/in/nigelkbishop

"Succinct points and clear advice in a neat package. If you are setting up your business this book tells you clearly the issues you face and how to start dealing with them. Reading this business book in my second

year of trading, it was very interesting to realise just how important it is to get the fundamentals right from the beginning. Great advice succinctly put, this guide sets out a clear framework, checklist and where to go next. It is useful for setting up any kind of business."
CATH TAJIMA-POWELL, Arts & Heritage Project Manager
linkedin.com/pub/cath-tajima-powell

"A very useful guide with lots of useful links to assist with research. I especially like the checklist at the back as there are so many things to consider when you are starting up a business that it's easy to miss key components."
KAYE CRITTELL, NEA Project Manager
Let's Do Business Group
http://www.letsdobusinessgroup.co.uk/

"Essential reading for anyone who wants to start their own business."
CHARLOTTE ELFDAHL, Founder of Rockville Lampshades
Winner of 'Tomorrow's Business Builders Award 2013'
www.homeofrockville.co.uk

Printed in Great Britain
by Amazon